Table of Contents

Dietary Strategies for Slowing and Preventing Alzheimer's Disease

Alzheimer's Diet and Nutrition Guide - Foods to Eat and Avoid

1. Introduction to Alzheimer's Disease and Nutrition

Diet, exercise, the support of family and friends, and social activities have all been suggested to help slow down the increase of beta-amyloid proteins in the brain – a typical sign of the progression of the disease. Research has found numerous reasons why people with a high intake of GM foods have a significant risk of getting Alzheimer's. As can be expected in a general food plan, the Alzheimer's Diet is not very specific. It encourages the intake of a variety of fruits and vegetables, with an emphasis on those that are high in vitamins and antioxidants. However, guidelines are also provided as to what a good nutrition plan should and should not include.

Excessive inflammation and free radical damage are two of the most likely factors implicated in Alzheimer's disease. While the predominating theory is that it occurs when unnatural beta-amyloid proteins cause plaque to accumulate in a person's brain, research has suggested that many other factors also come into play. The food you eat – and don't eat – plays a critical role in increasing or decreasing your risk of developing Alzheimer's disease. Alzheimer's asks for a unique attention to each person diagnosed with the disease, but that might have recurring symptoms or similar evolution. Although there is no guarantee when it comes to preventing a disease as complicated as Alzheimer's, there is also no harm in trying to lead a healthier life.

1.1. Understanding Alzheimer's Disease

There is no firm test to determine Alzheimer's, given it's primarily a diagnosis of exclusion grounded upon the elimination of alternative possibilities. Common tests include memory check and blood testing, though imaging scans and disease biomarker tests for the cerebrospinal fluid showcase more potential for identifying Alzheimer's from other forms of dementia. Myriad factors contribute to the development of Alzheimer's disease, such as genetics, lifestyle, and environmental aspects. Dementia and eating issues feed off each other: dementia increases the risk of a decline in physical health through malnutrition (although treating the nutritional difficulties present doesn't systematically slow disease progression) and malnutrition may make cognitive functioning worse, notably below a body mass index of 20. Even without weight loss, high malnutrition rates can be present. If a connection does exist, it is likely rooted in Alzheimer's impact on hormone levels and regulatory systems linked to hunger, body weight, and food intake, primarily involving ghrelin and leptin.

The symptoms of Alzheimer's disease, collectively known as dementia, encompass severe consequences for thinking, mood, and behavior. Among the early symptoms include short-term memory problems and inability to retain learned information. In general, logical reasoning and potentially motor function may be compromised in the short term, whereas in the long term, the ability to communicate and provide general tasks to oneself is impaired. Diseases behind elderly dementia have largely been linked to Alzheimer's disease, a progressive brain disorder and the most common cause of dementia. The disease typically begins in later adulthood before accelerating post-diagnosis until death.

1.2. The Role of Nutrition in Alzheimer's Disease

In addition to the perfect diet that mitigates the risk of developing Alzheimer's, there is emerging research on dietary strategies that can influence the progression of the disease in individuals already diagnosed. These dietary strategies are especially important in the absence of disease-modifying drug treatments. As there is no uniform treatment for different kinds and stages of cognitive impairment and dementia, every person should get personalized dietary recommendations from their healthcare provider depending also on any other pre-existing health conditions. In general, diets of individuals living with dementia need to be rich in nutrients and energy – such as unsaturated instead of saturated fatty acids, fresh instead of processed food, complex instead of simple sugars - and aimed at protecting body weight, growing muscles, and filling up the glycogen reserves.

Nutrition and diet play a substantial role in health and wellbeing and can significantly influence the development and progression of various diseases and conditions. In Alzheimer's disease, evidence is increasingly pointing to the influence of dietary patterns and food choices on cognitive health and the course of the disease. At the same time, the brain's nutritional profile can be influenced by what we eat, and certain components in food and the quantities they're consumed can have a major impact on disease progression. As such, nutritional recommendations for both the general population and especially for individuals with Alzheimer's are becoming an increasingly popular subject in research.

2. Nutritional Guidelines for Alzheimer's Patients

Macronutrient criteria are based on an approach of 55-25-20 with carbohydrates, proteins, fats to provide a balanced dietary allowance covering amino acids, carbohydrates, and fats with antioxidant effect. High amounts of DHA and EPA in oily fish are associated with a decreased incidence of both pathological and physiological Alzheimer's; however, the American Alzheimer's Association cautions against eating fish with "high mercury or other toxins multiple times a week". Carbohydrate-rich foods include vegetables and fruits. A high intake of red and processed meat, vitamins necessary for brain health such as vitamin B12 and iron. As Alzheimer's progresses, Alzheimer's patients should drink a minimum of 7-8 cups or 1.7 to 2 kg of water per day, more during hot weather or exercise. Drink to forget to drink or during the day. Residents need a minimum of 1,500-1,600 mg of calcium and 40 IU of Vitamin D.

To ensure the best quality of life, Alzheimer's patients with a decreased appetite and nutritional intake may require altered dietary intake as their disease progresses. Since the brain cells of Alzheimer's patients do not function well, they may need fewer calories, but some patients may need more to maintain a healthy weight. Dietary guidelines for people with Alzheimer's focus on special dietary needs, meal planning, and food items for the recommended "brain-healthy" diet. A diet meeting Alzheimer's dietary standards provides vitamins and minerals, a balance of carbohydrates, protein, and fat, and plenty of water. Dehydration is increased in Alzheimer's due to forgetfulness and difficulty swallowing or chewing. The cells in the body are also sensitive to insulin resistance that may be caused by the Alzheimer's process, affecting the tissues and organs, so it is necessary to balance appropriate diet, physical activity with good sleep and relaxation. Alzheimer's alters the senses, taste and smell, so it is necessary to change texture or flavors, use extra protein and add different colors and textures with the food you provide. Caloric intake should be determined by calorie requirements, physical activity, and stage of dementia. Most patients need between 2,000-2,500 calories per day.

2.1. Caloric Intake and Energy Needs

Although many people start a diet when they first start to notice dementia symptoms, food intake is sufficient. At most, they just have to adjust the amount of food already eaten to their energy needs. We must absolutely avoid foods that are too oily or based on oil, such as fried food, as well as too spicy and/or extravagant dishes, especially in too large quantities, as they can cause problems or simply the patient does not wish to eat them. It is also important to ensure an adequate intake of minerals and vitamins, namely calcium, iodine, iron, selenium, and fluorine, as well as vitamins such as C and D. It is important to provide through the diet the principles that the body cannot synthesize alone. To reduce the risk of osteoporosis and bowel cancer, it is recommended to stimulate milk and dairy product consumption (3-4 times a day).

Maintaining an adequate energy level will ensure that the individual with Alzheimer's remains healthy and prevents them from accumulating tiredness and feelings of weakness. The caloric intake must be attuned to the individual's energy needs, which can be estimated based on their age and sex. The choice of foods to ensure this intake is set by increasing the consumption of foods that are usually good sources of energy and incorporating the use of added fats. Preference must be given to fruits, especially in a natural way. In this way, the therapeutic strategy will be oriented to ensure that the energy provided by food is maintained by adjusting dietary fat, in whole, significantly increasing Omega-3 consumption.

2.2. Macronutrients: Carbohydrates, Proteins, and Fats

In this section, we discuss the types of dietary energy-yielding compounds provided in foods. For each of these macronutrients - carbohydrates, proteins, and fats - we will touch on their importance in the management of Alzheimer's disease. Carbohydrates, proteins, and fats are our primary sources of energy and supply the necessary substrates for the synthesis of neurotransmitters, neurotrophins, cellular messengers, and support overall cognitive function. They also aid in the synthesis of hormones and in vitamin absorption. Furthermore, they help to maintain the body's nitrogen balance, support the production of antibodies, and break down nourished tissue. Carbohydrates, proteins, and fats should be consumed in a balanced amount to maintain general health and wellness. Without the required nutrients, it is difficult for you to adequately meet your nutritional requirements. Macronutrient intake contributes to a healthy mind and body, providing required energy as well as dietary balance, which supports the body's other activities by regulating hunger.

With a growing recognition of diet's importance, healthcare professionals are now more likely to include dietary guidance as part of a comprehensive Alzheimer's management plan. This trend reflects a broader shift within healthcare toward using preventive or therapeutic nutritional strategies. Patients, caregivers, and healthcare providers can then work together to design eating plans that help them maintain health and wellness. An evidence-based review of the nutrition-related effects of nutrient-specific and customized diets is presented here, with particular attention to Alzheimer's Disease and Related Dementias (ADRD).

2.3. Micronutrients: Vitamins and Minerals

The table is a summary based on different research outcomes. Hopefully, it provides clarity about ways to manipulate a person's overall diet in people with Alzheimer's in relation to having more cognitive decline through intake of different vitamins and minerals. This is a special kind of fat, mainly found in meat. The effect of this fat on a person's memory and thinking skills is unclear. In order to optimize your brain health, try to eat at least 3 grams of omega-3 (DHA and EPA) every week. This is especially important if you have already established some form of cognitive decline. You can eat omega-3 fats from different fish like mackerel, sardines, and salmon. You can also consume omega-3 (DHA and EPA) in fortified food.

In general, vitamins and minerals, also referred to as micronutrients, are really important for the body's normal growth and development. Through this process, they can also support the functioning of major systems in the body such as the cardiovascular system and the brain. Brain health is mainly dependent on a number of vitamins and minerals. For that reason, there is large research that aims to understand the relationship between taking in these specific vitamins, minerals, and overall diet quality and the constantly changing cognitive decline. As of now, there is increasing interest in finding out to what extent our diet in terms of vitamins and minerals can be manipulated to support brain health decline. This is particularly important in people with Alzheimer's, who will have other aspects of

their brain function being altered, possibly due to the aging
process.

Micronutrients - Vitamins and Minerals

2.4. Hydration and Fluid Intake

How much fluid is required? A person with Alzheimer's should drink eight 8-ounce glasses of water per day (or 2 liters) to stay properly hydrated. Urine color, as well as thirst, is a simple way to assess if adequate fluids are being consumed, especially for individuals who do not tend to experience thirst. Hydration can also be improved by drinking at regular intervals and sipping throughout the day, rather than trying to drink the entire daily water requirement in one go. Animal milk may also be drunk rather than water. Non-caffeinated drinks such as vegetable, chicken or beef broth, carbonated water, milk, juice, gelatin desserts, and popsicles may also count. Certain fruits and vegetables also offer hydration, such as melons, cucumbers, oranges, and lettuce leaves. It is important that fluids are offered in a manner that is familiar and convenient to the person.

Keeping hydrated is one of the most important aspects of nutritional care in individuals with Alzheimer's disease. Alzheimer's patients at all stages are at an increased risk of dehydration due to disruptions in the brain that prevent the feeling of thirst. They may also have difficulty finding or accessing drinks, may forget to drink, and may struggle with swallowing. Even mild dehydration can affect cognitive function, causing disorientation, dizziness, and confusion. At worst, dehydration can lead to heart arrhythmias, a drop in blood pressure, fever, or kidney problems, which may require hospitalization. Proper hydration can improve overall health, decrease stress, and provide more opportunities for communication for an Alzheimer's patient. This is an essential aspect of their care that should not be overlooked.

3. Foods to Include in an Alzheimer's Diet

Nuts and seeds are an excellent source of protein and packed with good fats. They contain omega-3 fatty acids which are very good for the brain. Choose unsalted and roasted to avoid extra sodium. Walnuts are especially good for the brain. Many people have compared walnuts to the appearance and structure of the brain. They play a critical role in protecting cognitive function including learning and memory. Blackberries are full of vitamins and fiber and rich in antioxidants which can also protect against stress. Antioxidants help us get oxygen to our brains. Just like fruits and veggies, whole grains are packed with antioxidants and are excellent for brain functioning. They are also loaded with fiber and healthy fats. Dark leafy greens such as collards, spinach, kale, and arugula are rich in vitamins C, A, and K, together with plenty of iron and calcium. Spinach is linked to more success with long-term brain health. Sweet potatoes got a bad rap as being unhealthy but they are wonderful for the brain. The vitamins, antioxidants, the color comes from beta-carotene which is converted to vitamin A, including vitamins A, K, B6, manganese, magnesium, and vitamin C that studies show also help in improving cognitive decline and maintaining brain functioning. Most don't consider beans brain foods but they are very high in fiber, loaded with vitamins, potassium, copper, iron, and magnesium. Beans can also help reduce the risk of coronary artery disease.

Choosing foods for improving Alzheimer's symptoms must be done with extreme care and planning. Use this guide to find a meal plan that suits your loved one's preferences and remember to seek advice from a healthcare professional regarding individual dietary adjustments. Some of the best brain foods to prevent Alzheimer's disease are lean proteins like legumes, eggs, and fish, vegetables rich in vitamins, antioxidants, and healthy fats, fresh fruit, leafy greens, and nuts.

3.1. Fruits and Vegetables

Though limited, some studies suggest that higher intakes of antioxidant vitamins (such as C, E, and beta-carotene, a form of vitamin A) have been associated with lower dementia risk. Other Alzheimer's-protective fat-soluble vitamins that can be obtained through the regular consumption of vitamin-rich, bright, and dark-colored fruits and vegetables include vitamin C (an antioxidant thought to help maintain healthy cognitive function), vitamin E (improves cognition and brain health), and vitamin K. Additionally, recently published scientific research suggests that one of the vitamin B variants, niacin (a form of vitamin B3), when combined with other healthy lifestyle factors and dietary choices, such as the regular consumption of fresh fruit, vegetables, and whole grains, may protect against some of the well-known cellular hallmarks associated with Alzheimer's disease. In Alzheimer's-style dementia, niacin transportation into cells in the brain may be impaired; higher intakes found in whole foods, it is suggested, may supply enough to help prevent phosphate build-ups in neurons, which are considered one of the earliest signs of this dementia.

A diet comprised of nutrient-dense foods can be beneficial for individuals with Alzheimer's, supporting overall health and functioning as well as brain health. Whether consumed raw, cooked, or juiced, fruits and vegetables are high in essential nutrients such as vitamin C and dietary fiber, and antioxidants, which can help reduce cellular inflammation in the body, thereby improving health. Though controversial and largely unsupported by research, some scientists believe that vitamins and antioxidants can help to shield, repair, and rejuvenate nerve cells (neurons) and brain cells, thereby promoting longevity and protecting against cognitive decline. Preliminary research in small groups has also suggested that some vitamins found in fruits and vegetables may delay the onset of Alzheimer's in healthy older adults, though not in persons who already had the disease. However, no food, combination of foods, or dietary supplements can cure or prevent dementia or Alzheimer's disease, research indicates, regardless of the evidence of protective health benefits these foods may offer when included in a well-rounded, healthy diet.

3.2. Whole Grains

The nutritional profile that the brain can profit from is represented by certain grains. By supplying us with energy, they help us focus on our everyday activities and pay attention. Our memory is supported by building the myelin sheath—a protective protein cover around the nerves in our brains that enables our memory to pass more quickly by forming these nutritious fats. Gluten intolerance or celiac disease when opting for meals can prevent incorporating grains. Gluten is also present in oats, but the type present in oats doesn't normally affect individuals with a certain level of gluten sensitivity. Even provided that whole grains contain nutritious fiber, people may need to continue consuming as they usually did rather than adding foodstuffs with extreme fiber such as barley since 20 or more grams may not be tolerated by certain individuals.

The body can benefit from whole grains, which are carbohydrates containing essential fats and proteins, as well as vitamins B and E. They also contain calcium, iron, and magnesium, with dietary fiber present too. This combination of nutrients can lower cholesterol levels. Dietary fiber has the added benefits of enhancing digestion and stopping constipation. 100 percent whole wheat bread, muffins, and bagels alongside bran cereals, brown rice, and oatmeal are all options for incorporating more whole grains into the diet. Alzheimer's patients can obtain most or all of the 25 grams of fiber required every day by consuming these. Without frying them in unhealthy oils, meals can further incorporate whole grains.

3.3. Healthy Fats: Omega-3 Fatty Acids

The extent of the brain benefits of omega-3 fatty acids is still being scientifically investigated, but it's theorized that DHA is the most important property for brain health. Eating fatty fish, a key dietary source of DHA, has been found to be supportive of brain health. For example, a study appearing in JAMA documented that in adults without dementia but with memory complaints, relatively minimal fish intake - an average of just 1.3 servings per week - was associated with delays in the onset of decline in some cognitive and functional brain measures compared with no seafood consumption. According to a study published in the Journal of the American Medical Association, having at least one serving of fish (particularly fatty fish) per week or greater than one serving of each type of fish per month was associated with a slower decline in cognitive function.

Omega-3 fatty acids, commonly found in fatty fish but also in certain nuts and seeds (especially flaxseeds and walnuts) and plant oils such as flaxseed oil and canola oil, are considered to be healthy fats with a host of wide-ranging health benefits including their anti-inflammatory effects. But when it comes to Alzheimer's diet and nutrition, the omega-3 fatty acids available from fatty fish are credited with being of particular benefit for brain health, including supporting memory, speed of processing, and cognitive function among those with pre-clinical or early stages of Alzheimer's. Docosahexaenoic acid (DHA), one of the two omega-3 fatty acids found in the brain, makes up between 15 percent and 20 percent of the brain's cerebral cortex, the part of the brain responsible for memory, thinking, understanding, and reasoning, signaling DHA's potential link to improving cognitive function.

Be sure to avoid or limit cuts of meat that are higher on the fat scale such as rib-eye, T-bone, full-cut steaks, chuck, round, bottom sirloin, flank steak, hot dogs, sausage, and marbled, wagyu, bison, and kobe. Pay attention to preparation techniques and portion sizes as these can impact how healthy and lean the protein is. Grilling, roasting in the oven, searing, and braising are preferred methods. When pan-frying is necessary due to preference, use as little fat as possible and remove excess fat from the meat. Instead of deep frying things like pieces of chicken or fish, try 'oven frying' by using things like panko or unsweetened shredded coconut to create a crust. Fish can be a great source of lean protein. Healthy fish include wild pink and Sockeye salmon, tuna, and halibut. It is recommended to avoid shark, swordfish, king mackerel, white albacore tuna, big eye tuna, Spanish albacore, and tilefish.

Protein is found in foods that contain fish, eggs, poultry (e.g. chicken, turkey, quail, duck, and goose), pork (e.g. tenderloin, loins, sirloin, and ham), and lean cuts of beef and game meats (e.g. tenderloin, sirloin, and loin). These lean proteins can be a very important part of the diet for a person living with Alzheimer's or any dementia as it is important for individuals' muscles. When looking at a menu and choosing a protein for a meal, think about how the individual with dementia eats the proteins. If they can hold a fork, try a small grilled chicken breast, scrambled eggs, or a hamburger slider. If they may not be able to hold a fork, try protein that can be served with a spoon such as a good quality thick fish (e.g. salmon, swordfish, tuna, Atlantic cod, etc.), chili vom Fass, beef stew, lamb stew, lamb & rice hot dish, ground beef belly bombers with gravy, egg-based casseroles, chicken pot stickers with sauce, Mongolian beef, or teriyaki meatballs.

3.5. Antioxidant-Rich Foods

Green leafy vegetables are a good choice because they are high in antioxidants, and they generally taste better if cooked, rather than raw. There's a whole myriad of antioxidants, which you can include in your diet, that benefit you in ways you can only imagine. Omega-3 fatty acids combined with antioxidants benefit brain function and have been shown to possess anti-inflammatory properties. They help minimize the toxic and inflammatory compounds in the brain, and, as an added bonus, can help lower your risk of developing several age-related chronic diseases such as dementia, heart disease, and stroke. Omega-3 fatty acids, including ALA, which feeds into DHA and EPA also, can be found in the following foods: walnuts, rap oil, algae oils, fish such as mackerel, salmon, and sardine, etc. Omega-3 fatty acids can also be obtained from a number of different supplements to support optimal brain health or replace a diet limiting in these fatty acids.

In research looking at chronic diseases such as neurodegenerative cognitive diseases and various cancers, incorporating foods that contain high quantities of antioxidants and have anti-inflammatory components fitting into the 'Mediterranean Diet' can promote brain health and overall lower body inflammation. Because a person living with Alzheimer's already has a degree of brain atrophy and inflammation, benefiting from antioxidant-rich foods at any stage of progression would be beneficial. Educating the caregiver and person living with Alzheimer's on antioxidants is a simple way to include foods that are helpful to a person's nutritional needs and dietary benefits. In a hale and hearty brain, antioxidants including vitamins A, C, E and elements such as selenium are present in the body fighting off the onslaught of harmful substances our bodies face every day. There are even more natural antioxidants that are viable such as vitamin C which is safe and essential for the body.

4. Foods to Avoid in an Alzheimer's Diet

Fermented or aged foods: Certain fermented or aged foods contain biogenic amines, including histamine, which could lead to sudden changes in behavior related to histamine intake. Histamine-rich foods include cheese, processed meats, and alcohol. Rotten eggs may also contain these toxic chemicals.

Foods that may contribute to high cholesterol levels: Avoid dairy products containing animal fats, trans fats, hydrogenated fats, and saturated fat. These include butter, cream, processed cheese, fried foods, and vegetable shortening. Although red meat, high-fat beef, and pork are high in protein, they also contain saturated fat, which can be harmful to a person with Alzheimer's. Fried foods are also high in the unhealthy kind of fats.

Sweets and high-sugar items: A person with Alzheimer's should cut down on or eliminate sweets. Their food and drinks should have little or no sugar.

Caffeinated drinks: Caffeine can have a diuretic effect, leading to an increased urination frequency. This in turn may result in dehydration. It's also a stimulant. It's best to cut back on drinks such as coffee, tea, carbonated/cola soft drinks, and cocoa.

It is necessary to avoid certain foods and beverages for a person with Alzheimer's disease as they could cause memory loss and hamper the effectiveness of medications being taken by the patient. Memory loss is a common symptom associated with the disease; therefore, it is important to follow a healthy and well-balanced Alzheimer's diet for maximum nutrition and better health. There are certain foods a person with Alzheimer's should avoid. This article highlights the foods to avoid in an Alzheimer's diet, with the hope that a family member or caregiver finds this information useful while planning meals for their loved one.

4.1. Saturated and Trans Fats

Individuals may reduce their intake of these fats by checking food labels when shopping for groceries and electing food items with lower amounts of them, usually finding healthier alternatives to the kinds of fats mentioned in fresh, unprocessed foods. Animal fats, for example, also found in egg yolks, can be replaced by plant fats derived from fruits such as avocados, nuts, and seeds. It is also recommended that individuals eat more fish due to the fish fats improving cardiovascular health and overall brain functioning. Chia seeds, walnuts, canola oil, and tofu count as other sources of these fats.

Saturated fats, which are mainly found in cheese, red meat, whole-fat dairy, and butter, often increase the "bad" cholesterol in the bodies, leading to the development of chronic conditions such as heart problems. Some studies have pinpointed a link between high consumption of these fats and worse cognitive function. Trans fats, which are another type of fat mostly found in baked goods, fried foods, and some margarine, are considered the most dangerous for cognitive performance and inflammation, as they also lower the levels of "good" cholesterol in the blood, replacing them with the more detrimental variants. For these reasons, it may be advisable for Alzheimer's disease patients to avoid or significantly reduce the intake of saturated and trans fats since these fats have a negative impact on cardiovascular health, which, in turn, brings harm to cognitive functioning. Still, evidence on the topic is not certain, and the World Health Organization goes as far as recommending replacing some intake of saturated and trans fats with unsaturated fats, be it monounsaturated or polyunsaturated, to help with risk factors for Alzheimer's disease.

4.2. Added Sugars and Sweetened Beverages

Reducing consumption of added sugars and sweetened beverages is relatively simple. As mentioned previously, when processed foods are eaten only on occasion, sugar intake is naturally minimized. The human body is well-equipped to deal with the sugars that occur naturally in whole foods. Drinking mainly water, consuming fewer sweetened beverages, and eating more fruit instead of sweets are other methods to moderate sugar usage. Artificial sweeteners have few caloric value and no effect on blood glucose, making them suitable for people with diabetes. However, the growing evidence on their negative health effects makes them an unattractive beverage and food additive from a brain health perspective.

Added sugars may have several adverse effects on your cognitive well-being. For instance, added sugars encourage the production of cytokines - small proteins which regulate inflammation. Higher levels of some cytokines have been found in the blood of both Alzheimer's patients and overweight individuals in general. They can also increase oxidative stress, which is another mechanism implicated in Alzheimer's. Sugar can also lower the neurotransmitter brain-derived neurotrophic factor (BDNF), the endogenous growth factor involved in memory capacity. Finally, the body's response to added sugars can promote additional inflammation and other mechanisms which may damage the brain.

4.3. Processed and Fried Foods

Deep-fried foods, such as French fries, potato chips, and fried chicken, should be limited or avoided in elders in general and Alzheimer's patients in particular. When cooking, try to bake, roast, broil, or grill instead of frying, as much as possible or consider using an air fryer. Following a Mediterranean diet, made up of nutrient-dense foods and healthy fats, can help preserve cognitive function. This diet can be beneficial to people with Alzheimer's. In this diet, healthful whole foods such as nuts, seeds, fruits, vegetables, healthy fats, whole grains, some dairy, legumes and beans, and in moderate amounts, fish, poultry, and red wine are consumed. Red meats and sweetened beverages need to be limited as much as possible.

It is widely known that processed foods can wreak havoc in the bodies of people, regardless of whether they suffer from any ailment or not. These foods, along with fried foods, are not mainly beneficial for Alzheimer's patients. The reasons are that these foods can potentially increase the levels of bad cholesterol, aggravate issues like diabetes, blood pressure, and gastrointestinal symptoms. In such situations, people with Alzheimer's should be encouraged to limit processed, canned, jarred, or pre-mixed food intake as far as possible.

4.4. High-Sodium Foods

STRATEGIES TO LIMIT HIGH-SODIUM FOODS. To lessen the significance of a high-sodium diet, and the potential for water retention, elevated blood pressure and an increased risk for chronic diseases, the following strategies can be incorporated. By taking the time to read the ingredients label of pre-packaged food, have a general understanding of ingredients that are higher in sodium, shopping for lower sodium products and using it instead of the original ingredient, using alternative seasonings and staying fortuned with fresh, easy ways to quickly cook balanced meals, a reduced sodium diet can be feasible for families affected by Alzheimer's. Consider prioritizing lower-sodium foods for some meals that are part of a healthy and active lifestyle, including breakfast or dinner. It may be easier for the individual with Alzheimer's to accept lower-sodium grains at breakfast, such as unflavored oatmeal or whole grain toast with unsalted margarine, rather than at dinner when nutrient-packed and lower-sodium rice, pasta or potato. It may be easier for the individual with Alzheimer's to accept lower-sodium veggies at lunch rather than for dinner when satisfying, lower-sodium and nutrient-packed veggies can help maintain a healthy weight and brain.

High-sodium foods. Skip high-sodium servings, which can raise blood pressure and dehydrate individuals. Herbal seasoning blends can replace salt in recipes and on foods. A dietary excess of one category of food that can have a negative affect on the brain is foods that contain high amounts of sodium, also known as table salt. A low-sodium food is defined as containing 140 milligrams or less of sodium per serving. High-sodium foods to reduce or eliminate from the Alzheimer's diet are canned, dehydrated, dried, and rehydrated foods, such as instant rice, instant oatmeal, flavored pasta, flavored rice, flavored side dishes; canned or dried soups, stews, chili, chowder. Only eat low-sodium or reduced sodium varieties of canned sauerkraut, tomatoes, vegetables or tomato sauce; canned and processed meats and fish; hot dogs; ham.

5. Meal Planning and Preparation Tips

Raw Organic Eggs – eat 1-3 every day. They are super easy on the digestive tract and contain critical choline and other brain-boosting lipids. Free-range are typically much better than regular (also called "flaxseed-fed" eggs). Free ranging makes them more nutritious since the animal will be eating much more of their natural diet. Choline – in full doses like you will be achieving with 3-5 eggs a day, you are going to allow the body to help construct new brain cells, creating the stem cell fluid needed for cerebral fluid. Glutathione – found in the yolk, glutathione is one of the most powerful antioxidants in the body. It's rich in sulfur, critical for detoxifying the liver, as well as promoting healthy bile flow (1 of the 2 detoxification pathways your body needs in order to prevent neurotoxicity). Wild-caught Fish – all meat supplied to your loved one should be lower in metals, such as mercury. Wild-caught meat is lower in metals than fish from a farm. Mindful Meals - It is also important to stay present and enjoy your meals. Use these meals to build and strengthen the relationship you have with your loved one. Enjoy the connection and the time spent together, eating meals is not just about the food your loved one eats, it is about the company and the additional love these meals bring.

Sprinkle these incredible foods in and watch the brain health improve:

When creating your meal plans, keep food listed in this guide in mind as they are nutritionally powerful, full of powerful brain-boosting nutrients, and easy for many people in the later stages of Alzheimer's disease to eat. Below are some tips for getting the nutrients needed to fight Alzheimer's disease into meals and planning them for your loved one.

5.1. Creating Balanced Meals

Offer regular, balanced snacks. People with Alzheimer's disease may experience "sundowning." Often, as the day wears on, their appetite decreases. If they eat large meals, they may be less hungry at the next meal. Offering regular small meals and snacks throughout the day gives them the opportunity to eat a balanced diet. This will help to maintain their overall health and provide the necessary vitamins and minerals to sustain strength and resistance. Avoid serving snacks too close to mealtime; it could spoil their appetite. Adding small portions of meat, fruit or vegetables, and a piece of cheese, bread, fruit, or a dessert provides a nice combination. Cooking and shopping for nutritional food can be a challenge for caregivers. Many foods that are easy to prepare are unhealthy and don't provide the nutrients a body needs. Planning is the key to being successful.

Creating balanced meals Balanced meals are crucial in maintaining the health of people with Alzheimer's disease. When serving a meal, make sure it is balanced. Balance means that meals are nutritious and contain foods from all the food groups in the Food Pyramid. This will help provide the vitamins and minerals needed to maintain strength and endurance. While people with Alzheimer's disease are different, all individuals benefit from balance.

Nutritious meals can help to maintain a person's overall health and improve their quality of life, but serving them can be a challenge. Health conditions, medication side effects, dental problems, and Alzheimer's disease are just a few of the reasons why appetite decreases and eating habits can change.

5.2. Adapting Recipes for Alzheimer's Patients

When it comes to how we actually scale down our ingredients, we first make our recipes according to the product information provided by those who own and distribute the pieces we are using. If "Company XYZ" states that their saucepan usually produces 12 portions as the recipe is cooked, we make dishes that we enjoy for our families at home all of a sudden have 6 easy servings that are "full dish." When we get to the cooking phase of each recipe, we separate all into two neat containers.

Smaller items or chopped or cut up items. Keep everything expected in meals tiny, especially when it comes to vegetables and meats. We find that even those who initially object to this rule eventually accept the change. We might still hear a loved one complaining of not having enough food seconds later. Waterless and slow-cookers. Many seniors like slow-cookers since they produce soft food that is well-cooked. Meals on the ground. Sometimes it's difficult for people with Alzheimer's to use utensils, so make the process easier by making "meals on the ground." Don't make any food, like grains or proteins, too prominent.

When you are preparing food for a loved one with AD or a form of dementia and are modifying food based on the current Alzheimer's diet, these general guidelines and ideas will help you to create the best meals. The important thing here is to meet the dietary needs of the person with

AD as closely as possible in whatever new recipes you come across.

ADAPTING RECIPES FOR COGNITIVE HEALTH

For many caregivers, the interaction that leaves the greatest impression on them is the flummoxed loved one standing in the kitchen wondering what they're doing...or not doing. If you're planning an Alzheimer's diet today, whether for any of the stages of Alzheimer's or just to eat healthier and improve cognitive function, take the following guidelines into account.

5.3. Mealtime Strategies

Another idea is to replace a vanilla supplement in the evening with a fruit shake using chocolate flavored protein powder. The combination of supper and the sweet treat may help the person feel satisfied and full.

Individuals all need some 'me' time before sharing a meal; Follow the person's wishes about eating can help make meals special. Alzheimer's disease also affects appetite. One strategy is to cut back main courses and increase snacks. With a full plate an individual may forget to eat, but he or she is more likely to eat something small. Protein is the most often declined from the individual's normal meal. Protein is very important so it is important to provide small, high protein snacks that the individual likes. Be creative. What does the individual like to eat that is high protein? Examples may include a hard-boiled egg, small portion of chicken salad, etc.

Some other mealtime strategies include: Creating a calm, familiar environment; Plan regular meals—people often feel best following routines; Breakfast is a good time for meals for many individuals—people are often more alert in the morning; Are personality or cultural issues important in how someone eats a meal?

In enhancing food intake, one step may be to set aside times for the individual to remember to eat. Others may need to be prompted to eat during meals. Think of a strategy to help someone remember when it is time to eat or ask the person if he or she is hungry.

Strategy I: What are some mealtime strategies for an individual with Alzheimer's? What are the main strategies one can do to help an individual with Alzheimer's eat? Many individuals with Alzheimer's experience frustration during meals. These strategies may sound very simple, depending on how advanced the illness is, an individual with Alzheimer's may forget that they need to eat.

6. Special Considerations for Alzheimer's Patients

Alzheimer's disease is the most catastrophic emotional and financial ailment. This form of dementia has no cure, but the food you eat may help you keep dementia at bay. However, some pharmaceutical substances may decrease the power of your Alzheimer's medication or worsen symptoms. Be cautious of supplement use. Nutritional supplements should be discussed with your physician as there are many that interact with your medications and may decrease their effectiveness. Sugar should be monitored in clients affected by both diabetes and Alzheimer's disease. Some individuals with Alzheimer's disease may alter and become more aggressive if they consume sugar. It's critical to keep a comprehensive record of how your loved one reacts to certain foods or substances. If you believe any dietary modification has worsened their condition, notify their physician.

1. Some people with Alzheimer's disease may have difficulty with chewing and swallowing. Small amounts of food at a time and thoroughly cooking foods are simple ways to make food more palatable. 2. Some people with Alzheimer's disease may lose weight and others may gain. Try serving smaller portions of nutrient-rich foods and also high-calorie food like cookies and brownies to help with weight gains. 3. Some people with Alzheimer's disease may not drink enough fluids. Adequate fluid is essential in

maintaining good health. Some ways to encourage fluids is to make them more appealing.

Nutrition and eating involve special considerations for an individual with Alzheimer's disease. Poor appetite, swallowing difficulties, and lack of fluid intake are some of the most common challenges, along with the fact that food may not appear as tasty to someone with Alzheimer's. The person with Alzheimer's may lose some of their sense of taste and smell. The following are some things to keep in mind when it comes to feeding a person with Alzheimer's:

6.1. Chewing and Swallowing Difficulties

• Offer simple foods which are naturally in small parts ready for eating (like fruit and yogurt), or foods that crumble easily in the mouth. People with dementia usually require fewer calories, so making sure they eat healthier foods can be beneficial. For example, the individual may drink a butter and nuts smoothie instead of consuming an almond-filled croissant. • Modify the meals so that they are easier to handle. Half a sandwich may get less difficult to eat than a long plate with food on it. Reducing the number of course in a meal can also help. • Change the mealtimes to fit the patient with Alzheimer's usual day; those who are most active in the late afternoon are the most likely to eat a bigger meal in the afternoon than in the morning. • Creativeness by making it interesting and developing a nice dining atmosphere; try using plates of appealing colours for well-differentiated foods and cutlery that is weighted. • Offer enough fluid; certain people have a difficult time swallowing liquids. Drive away from thin liquids like area and offer options that are more comfortable and appealing. Following each gulp, some individuals may enjoy eating a slice of lemon or mango. • Minimal chewing, especially when it comes to food. A person having a minor difficulty in swallow should consume pureed/smoothed food because less effort is needed to swallow it. • Decrease the number of frequency of solids or whatever is problematic for the patient to chew safely; for instance, infant dishes, ironed bowls or a rice/plant mix.

About one-third of nursing home residents suffer from chewing or swallowing problems, as the mechanisms for the two activities are closely linked. Additionally, more than 60% of all elderly possess age-induced dysphagia disorders. It is not infrequent for these problems to occur in connection with the presence of other health issues. Thus, persons with Alzheimer's often suffer from difficulties in swallowing. These difficulties can increase the risk of sucking and breathing at the same time. Difficulties during swallowing can easily lead to feelings of fear and anxiety in persons affected by the illness. As food often ends up in the lungs rather than the stomach, a coughing reflex might be triggered due to the inconsistency of food. Even the voice can become hoarser and the tongue can be paralyzed. To prevent this, the mouth should be closed when swallowing, which is why those affected by Alzheimer's often find it hard to breathe. Fortunately, however, the swallowing reflex itself is not usually affected. It is just that the feedback from the brain of someone affected by Alzheimer's does not always let them know how they are meant to swallow, which can frequently result in vomiting. Here are a few tips to make chewing and swallowing easier and to reduce the danger of getting food stuck in one's throat.

6.2. Weight Management

If there is any suspicion that a person with Alzheimer's disease is not eating, a daily food diary for 3-7 days that includes portion size can provide invaluable evidence for problem-solving changes. Regular biweekly weight checks and monitoring of food and water intake with a daily or weekly checklist of risks for eating and drinking problems or risks can also be completed. Referral to a registered dietitian for an assessment and advice on improvement of diet and increasing food intake is essential. It is important to note that family and healthcare professionals should never force a person with Alzheimer's disease to eat as a first-line treatment. It is critical to recognize and manage a decrease in food intake as part of the disease process rather than something within a person's control or likely to be amenable to a quick fix.

Current guidelines for the management of dementia and other neurological disorders in people with mild cognitive impairment and early-stage Alzheimer's disease strongly encourage the maintenance of a healthy body weight, without any rapid, involuntary weight loss. They recommend monitoring food and water intake and weight on a bi-weekly basis to optimize intake and avoid any unusual decline in caloric intake, water intake, or weight change. Eating disorders such as food refusal, anorexia, hyperphagia, and severe weight loss can dramatically impact disease progression and mortality. Reduced appetite can lead to insufficient vitamin and mineral intake which can further impact medications, like for example, the antipsychotic drugs used to treat severe neuropsychiatric symptoms not responding to nonpharmacological interventions. Deficits can further lead to poor muscle mass, called sarcopenia, which increases the risk of falls and impact daily functionality more than just being underweight.

6.3. Medication Interactions

If a loved one is on a medication regimen and taking
Alzheimer's supplements, find out if there are any dietary
components that they should avoid or other considerations
that should be taken into account. Caregivers also need to
know if they should wait two hours after a dose to give any
nutritional supplements such as Alzheimer's vitamins or
brain health supplements. Likewise, if a loved one should
take their Alzheimer's supplement with a meal, caregivers
need to know and should also be informed when the
supplement should be taken. Do not be shy about asking
questions for the safe administration of the medication.

Diet and medication

Alzheimer's disease has a wide range of symptoms and it's
highly variable from person to person. For this reason, it's
critical to manage diet and diet composition and entrust
the medication regimen into the care of a healthcare
professional or other qualified experts.

Diet and diet composition

When someone with Alzheimer's disease is taking certain
medications, the foods they eat can interact with the
medications. This can lead to side effects, problems with
the effectiveness of the medication, or other issues.
Alzheimer's caregivers administering care at home need to
also be aware of these food and medication interactions.
Healthcare professionals involved in care management

should also take potential food and medication interactions into account.

Diet and nutrition issues to consider when taking medication

7. The Importance of Regular Exercise

It is recommended that you check with your doctor before starting any exercise routine. It is also recommended to do the exercise correctly and in a safe place. Do an exercise that can be done together and has acquired standard education about these exercises, especially for those who have mobility constraints. All exercises are proof of total care for one's own body while carrying out any of these activities. Not only increase strength and mobility, but also can improve the atmosphere which can reduce the frequency of difficult behaviors such as continuous calls, asking the same questions, or walking for a while. If necessary and after an assessment by a doctor, people with Alzheimer's can include difficult or special activities in progressive sports or rehabilitation programs.

Experts recommend that they exercise for at least 150 minutes per week. The exercise carried out is varied every day. According to the U.S. National Institute on Aging, the best kind of exercise is endurance exercise. Because it can benefit the cardiovascular, the ability of the lungs, and the heart and prevent some diseases from occurring. Not only that, but exercises also provide many benefits such as reducing the risk of depression, stress, and anxiety. That is why people who have Alzheimer's disease or any other dementia should do exercises regularly. Because essentially all that is good for the heart is also good for the brain. It can reduce the likelihood of cognitive decline. Also, do a variety of exercises that can be done to reduce pain, reduce the risk of headaches, and prevent the loss of abilities to perform daily activities. Exercises can also help the medicines for dementia to be more effective in improving memory and thinking skills, especially that obtained from resistant exercises.

We are aware that currently, there is no cure for Alzheimer's. Also, there is no treatment that stops or slows its progress, but it is important for some activities and care to relieve those suffering from Alzheimer's. Regular physical activity is an important goal to achieve the best quality of life in patients with Alzheimer's disease. A person with Alzheimer's can do various activities so that their body strength can be maintained. Starting from gardening, yoga, aerobics, cycling, and many more. For a person with Alzheimer's disease, some light exercises can also have tremendous benefits. Exercises that are automatically performed as part of everyday life can also help maintain or improve physical and mental health.

7.1. Physical Benefits of Exercise

- One set of sit-to-stands: have the individual with Alzheimer's sit in a non-padded armchair with his/her feet shoulder-width apart and flat on the ground. Guard the person's body as he/she rises up to a standing position and then sits back down. Perform repetitions as appropriate. - One seated-stands exercise: from the chair, have the individual with Alzheimer's stand using a walker, making certain the walker is stable before having the person proceed to walk.

To obtain these benefits, the individual with Alzheimer's should engage in the following routine ten to twelve times per day:

- Improved strength: Regular physical activity enhances muscle strength and endurance, increasing overall physical capacity and delaying the progression of Alzheimer's symptoms. - Mobility: Regular strength training and exercise can help the individual with Alzheimer's maintain mobility for a longer period of time. - Overall Health: Besides the positive impact on cognitive function, physical activity is good for cardiovascular health, bone density, blood pressure, diabetes, depression, and eating habits. It also can contribute to weight loss or maintenance. - Biologic benefits: According to research, physical activity stimulates the development of new brain cells and can slow mental decay.

Engagement in regular physical exercise will provide the following physical benefits to people with Alzheimer's disease:

------------------------- 7.1. Physical Benefits of Exercise -------------------------

7.2. Mental and Emotional Benefits

The general feeling is that a social or group setting is good for promoting fun and motivation (will have a longer commitment to attending) and is also good for cognitive health. Because the cognitive function and memory may continue to decline and is unlikely to be reversed, exercise professionals have focused more attention on the emotional benefits of exercise for the population. Mental illness can occur due to Alzheimer's, depression, and anxiety are common and can harm the quality of life. Depression can hurt these stressors by decreasing internal resources, especially to deal with the daily difficulties of the family member's ability to do things on their own, and so on.

Exercisers in general tend to be less anxious, angry, or depressed than non-exercisers, and today's exercise may, in effect, improve mood for a few hours after exercising. Through talking with the caregivers, we discovered a handful of small behavioral changes called "Sundowning." This group became convinced that the best form of exercise takes place when a person with Alzheimer's is performed is caregiver-led exercise in a small group setting. Short sessions at a level that is high enough to lead to healthy fatigue incorporate different types of exercise (strength, aerobic balance, flexibility, coordination).

Physical activity has many mental and emotional benefits for people with Alzheimer's. It can improve cognitive functioning in people with mild memory problems and may slow the progression to full-fledged Alzheimer's disease. For people with more advanced memory loss, physical activity can decrease depression and anxiety, both direct side effects of Alzheimer's, and neurological. People who have been physically active throughout their lives tend to do better with Alzheimer's disease than those who were sedentary, and they function for a longer time as their disease progresses.

8. Nutrition and Brain Health Research

Interventions to date include dietary outcomes that target brain function and have coupled effects on mental health and wellbeing. The relationship between diet and Alzheimer's and other dementias is still mostly uncertain, especially given the lack of effective treatment for the condition. Consequently, much of the research suggestive of diet's potential role in Alzheimer's are grounds for ongoing exploration. It is important to note that this topic of research is continuously evolving as studies generate new insights into diet and brain health. This may be useful to caregivers or family members of individuals with Alzheimer's; healthcare professionals who offer dietary advice; and researchers who have an interest in the findings for nutritional determinants of brain health.

The role of nutrition in brain health has gained increasing attention in the research community over the past two decades. Early studies focused on specific nutrients and links to brain health, but recent efforts have expanded to include dietary patterns. A growing body of scientific evidence now supports the idea that nutrients and overall diet are linked with cognitive function. There are several programs and projects underway trying to determine the most appropriate approach to studying diet and cognition, including the development of new questionnaires, as well as stand-alone databases and repositories. Global efforts have launched specific guidelines or public health updates related to nutrition and dementia, which includes standard recommendations for maintaining a healthy diet.

8.1. Studies on Diet and Cognitive Function

None of these studies are specific to Alzheimer's disease. Nonetheless, a balanced and varied diet appears likely to be brain-protective and to reduce the risks of developing an age-related, dementing process such as AD. In the intervening period, when symptoms of an incipient AD have developed to a clinically diagnosable level, diet remains very important and can help with the management of complications associated with the condition, as well as playing a role in general health maintenance. The following dietary considerations consider values and deficiencies in the context of care for someone diagnosed with probable AD, and not just the reduction of dementia risk.

Recent years have seen increasing interest in the concept of the "food-brain axis," exploring the relationship between diet and cognitive function. Evidence from these studies suggests that poor nutrition has a negative impact on brain health, while dietary improvement yields cognitive advantages. Influential longitudinal studies like the Whitehall II Study showed that a diet abundant in fruit, vegetables, and fish was associated with reduced cognitive decline. Additionally, the 5-year FINGER study reported that an improved, Mediterranean-style diet was associated with better cognitive function. Other meta-analyses have suggested undernutrition is associated with impaired cognitive function. However, given the diverse ethical issues and methodological considerations relevant to studies of diet and cognition, few important, hard facts have emerged.

8.2. Impact of Nutrition on Brain Health

A balanced diet may decrease low-grade inflammation in the brain that is associated with the development of neurodegenerative diseases, such as Alzheimer's disease. Malnutrition has been associated with accelerated cognitive decline. Research suggests that antioxidants can help maintain brain health, protect neurons, and reduce the symptoms of memory loss associated with Alzheimer's disease. Furthermore, the omega-3 polyunsaturated fatty acids (PUFAs) have been shown to have a protective influence on brain cells by slowing cell breakdown and increasing the protective chemical called Brain-Derived Neurotrophic Factor (BDNF). A study has shown in humans and animals to reduce deposits of the Alzheimer's protein beta-amyloid, which are designed to build up in the brain.

Dietary interventions or approaches can provide an effective means of supporting cognitive function and reducing the prevalence of some neurodegenerative conditions, although evidence is still emerging. Many believe that food doesn't only help us combat the chances of developing physical health issues but also brain diseases. Adequate nutrition is essential for brain function and overall health. Suboptimal nutritional status is associated with mental health problems and increased morbidity from neurodegenerative disorders. A diet high in saturated fats can increase production of harmful lipids which can damage neurons. Overproduction of free radicals released as by-products of energy metabolism in the brain can also damage brain cells. Additionally, unhealthy diets can increase the risk of neurodegenerative conditions through their effects on risk factors for physical health.

9. Practical Tips for Family Caregivers

Limit the options. If a person has difficulty making decisions, limit the number of food choices. Provide just one item at a time instead of offering two or more foods at once. Designate when meals and snacks will be served. Provide a structured meal time for the meals, approximately every four hours. Make foods easy to chew. People with Alzheimer's may have trouble chewing and swallowing. Grind or finely chop meats, fruits and vegetables to make them easier to eat. Offer alternatives to foods that require chewing. Use vitamins and supplements only if needed. Vitamins or supplements are not a replacement for a nutritious diet, but some individuals may need these products because of a chronic condition. Always consult a healthcare provider or registered dietitian nutritionist before providing any vitamin or supplements. Use special cups, plates and flatware. When food or liquid is easier to see, sometimes it's easier to consume. Inexpensive "nosey" cups and tableware specifically designed for Alzheimer's patients can be purchased online or at a hospital supply store.

In addition to tailoring foods to an individual's likes and dislikes, the following strategies can help you encourage a good diet in an Alzheimer's patient:

- Make a grocery list. Planning your week's meals in advance and making a list of items you need can make grocery shopping more efficient. - Shop for groceries when help is available. If possible, try to shop for groceries when you can leave your loved one with someone else. - Choose precooked or easy-to-prepare meals. While boxed, frozen or prepared food items are not always the healthiest option, they may be the easiest and quickest option for you. - Make leftovers for future meals. Consider the option of making a double recipe of your meals and freezing the leftovers to reheat later. - Set the table with simple place settings. Place a single setting of one utensil, napkin, and cup at each setting to maintain structure and aid with eating. - Break the meal into smaller courses. You may have better success if you serve the soup in a separate course from the entrée, and from the dessert. - Taste the food. Encourage your loved one to taste the food by saying, "This turned out well, why don't you try some?" - Provide feedback. Gently alert your loved one to consume food if they seem to be eating below a healthy caloric intake to prevent malnutrition.

Many caregivers find it difficult to navigate grocery shopping and meal preparation while attending to the needs of a loved one with Alzheimer's disease. However, these tasks can be simplified by following the tips listed below:

9.1. Grocery Shopping and Meal Preparation

Eating in a relaxed environment can assist with digestion and reduce the possibility of developing choking. Make foods that are high in iron, protein, and vitamin C if the person does not eat enough of them already. Iron-rich foods include red meat, eggs, pulses, and fortified breakfast cereals. Constipation can be particularly aggravating for the person with dementia. Aim for a bowel movement at least once a day. Offer plenty of fluids and dietary fibre, as found in such foods as whole meal bread, fruit and vegetables, flour. Use tinned fruit and add prune juice to the cottage pie. Healthcare professional specializing in dementia or a nutritionist can advise more on diet in these circumstances.

The most convenient option for providing appropriate food and drinks is to do grocery shopping and meal preparation for the week. In this case, it is more difficult to provide a variety of foods and meals that will satisfy the dietary needs of the person with dementia. As a general rule, the longer that the condition progresses, the more difficult it is to ensure that there is enough variety in the diet. Family carers can prepare and freeze meals in advance or make other long-life storage arrangements. Frozen vegetables and fruits are very useful, i.e., for soups and crumbles, casseroles. A person with dementia may eat better if you keep his or her meals simple, serve familiar food and drinks, thereby making eating more enjoyable; offer a wide variety of foods they enjoy; be patient and give the person plenty of time when eating.

9.2. Encouraging Healthy Eating Habits

Caring for someone with Alzheimer's can be challenging. Visit a registered dietitian (RD) for more detailed advice to create a meal plan that can help guide meal choices for people with Alzheimer's disease or dementia. They provide vitamins, minerals, energy-providing proteins, fats, and complex carbohydrates that are found in plant sources and other healthy foods. It is not practical to divide food into groups due to physical, cultural, or personal preferences. By working with the person with Alzheimer's likes and ensuring adequate and varied treats, you can create a nutritionally sound diet—all at moderate cost. Your wish to eat healthy is the most important. Work with the person when making decisions about their diets. Remember, what we eat can play a role in staying healthy.

Encouraging person-centered healthy eating habits for residents with dementia is an important aspect of nutrition care. I.G. provides a person-centered guide for creating positive eating experiences and for the overall promotion of nutritional health in individuals with Alzheimer's Disease or Related Dementia (ADRD). The following presents practical ways to plan for positive eating experiences for a person with Alzheimer's. First, however, are the foundations of a well-balanced diet plan for a person with Alzheimer's that are listed in your next communication.

9.3. Seeking Professional Guidance

In summary: Caregivers who are dealing with aging family members living at home and in long-term care programs will need to understand the necessary components of Alzheimer's nutrition and feeding a person with Alzheimer's. We have some starter information on our website and encourage you to follow the links listed in "The Facts of Alzheimer's Nutrition" section (see the left column of our web home page). Discussing these suggestions with a medical professional is also crucial. After looking over our information, would you like to talk with a professional about these concerns? If so, please provide us with your family member's contact information, so we can determine if our service will be beneficial.

Seek advice from a registered dietitian/nutritionist (RDN): Geriatricians and advanced practice nurses in the field of gerontology receive additional training in nutrition care issues specific to older adults. An RDN is more extensively trained in food and nutrition. Also, the RDN credential is regulated by the Commission on Dietetic Registration, so you can be assured when you find one that you are getting help from a food and nutrition expert. New Jersey Registered Dietitian/Nutritionist is the website where you can locate one.

Consult with healthcare professionals: If you are concerned with your loved one's eating habits, or if you have a senior citizen who is under an elder care program or assisted living program, turn to the doctor and registered dietitian/nutritionist in the facility for advice. Depending on your older adult's situation, the advice may vary.

Seek professional guidance: Your situation may differ from that of others. Seek help from your healthcare professional and a dietitian/nutritionist for the best solutions for your situation.

10. Resources for Further Information

Nutrition information: • The Academy of Nutrition and Dietetics maintains an online tool called Find an Expert. It is a listing of registered dietitians and/or nutritionists in your area. You can search for a professional who has worked extensively with people with Alzheimer's disease by entering "dementia care" and/or "Alzheimer's care" in the search area. • The USDA maintains an online tool called Supertracker. It enables you to make a basic dietary plan for yourself or someone else based on dietary needs, personal preferences, and a number of other health concerns, including Alzheimer's disease. Remember that Supertracker is designed for people with a normal BMI. See a calculator online at. If the person being planned for needs to gain weight or lose weight, talk with a knowledgeable professional, such as a registered dietitian or a nutritionist, who has caregiving experience.

General information for people with Alzheimer's disease and caregivers: • The Alzheimer Society • Alzheimer's Disease International • Alzheimer's Association • National Institute on Aging • The Alzheimer's Store • Caregiver Information about Dementia by Dr. Robert Bornstein

10.1. Alzheimer's Associations and Organizations

A list of Alzheimer's Associations and Organizations throughout Ontario and other information can be obtained by contacting the Alzheimer Society of Ontario at 4161 Old Kingston Road, Scarborough, Ontario, M1E 2M8. Tel. 416-398-8642 Toll-free 800-879-4226 E-mail: asinfo@alzheimerontario.com. Visit Methods 13. There is no cure for Alzheimer's disease, but treatments are available that focus on Alzheimer's for a copy of the document).

The following organizations and associations can help you with information and advice on this publication. Please contact them for further information on local support groups and local Community Care Access Centres in your area that are associated with the Alzheimer Society. These organizations and their services are free of charge. Remember, you are not alone. There are many people like you looking for answers and help. To download a copy of "Care Living with Alzheimer's, A workbook of information and resources," go to.

These local, national, and international organizations and associations can provide you with valuable support and information. They may provide funding for research and help direct you to possible sources for financial help. There is a wealth of information on other community-based services that can make living with Alzheimer's easier and inform you about the effect that the disease may have in the years ahead. In addition, they have a host of professionals that can help answer any questions you may have about care, services, or anything else concerning Alzheimer's.

10.2. Nutritionists and Dietitians

Nutrition professionals act according to ethical, personal, and cultural factors in order to make appropriate nutrition practices. Nutritionists and dietitians perform susceptible activities within the National Health Services in accordance with the laws and guidelines. Nutrition researchers have relationships with food science, health, and wellness sectors and they apply sound research principles and ethical standards. They use current evidenced-based protocols to counsel and guide individuals, families, extended health, and the public at large. They provide scientifically sound nutritional information and attend to the psychological factors that surround food choice. Based on the close relationship they have with the food and agricultural sectors, as well as health care providers, their codes of professional practice and scientific investigation necessarily follow.

Nutritionists and dietitians are very important for the AD patient because they provide advice on what to eat and what to avoid as far as diet is concerned. Nutritionists and dietitians develop eating plans tailored to the nutritional needs of a person with Alzheimer's disease. The meal plans are customized to a person's medical condition, medications, level of physical activity, and level of control over food intake. Family members and caregivers are taught how to help people with AD eat well and make sure they are drinking enough fluids. Nutrition professionals may recommend supplements if the patient's diet doesn't include elements that are important for nutrition and general health.

10.3. Online Tools and Apps

The search returned 17 tools and apps that met our inclusion criteria, reflecting a variety of functions, such as recipe inspiration and meal planning tools, trackers to monitor the intake of various nutrients and food composition databases. Many claimed to be designed for individuals with cognitive difficulties, although none had data to support these claims. All tools and apps are marketed for use by the general adult population. A meta-analysis has identified that nutrition-focused apps may be beneficial, potentially improving knowledge, attitudes, self-efficacy, and various health markers. However, in practice, only a very small proportion of people with Alzheimer's use any form of digital technology as a means of support, outside of social use. All respondents questioned at a public diet and dementia event had used the internet but had not accessed any dementia-specific apps and had no knowledge of what was available. Many of these participants were motivated by the shaped themes underpinning all guidance in the ENRICH framework.

In recognition of this, we have developed a series of 'Frequently Asked Questions', in collaboration with the Nutrition Group of the European Working Group of People with Dementia and ADI, answering the many questions that individuals with Alzheimer's, as well as their caregivers, might have about diet. As a rapidly evolving field, we are also mindful of the potential for technology to support the management of Alzheimer's and diet. We include in this document an up-to-date selection of freely available online tools and apps that are designed to support diet in various ways, aimed at interested individuals and caregivers as well as healthcare professionals.

Dietary Strategies for Slowing and Preventing Alzheimer's Disease

1. Introduction to Alzheimer's Disease and Nutrition

The following content reviews the neuropathology of Alzheimer's, the role of nutrition in its development, current dietary strategies that are associated with reduced risk for developing the disease or its associated dementia, current strategies being examined in intervention studies aimed at slowing progression of its associated brain changes or reversing the dementia already developing. A section which modifies one's nutritional habits can help to preserve mental health.

Alzheimer's disease affects millions worldwide, imposing a significant personal, medical, and financial burden. A major factor behind the growing prevalence of this condition is that average lifespan is increasing, allowing elderly people enough time to succumb to the disease. Because decades of degeneration of the brain precede clinical diagnosis of dementia, and dietary and physical activity risk factors have been identified, researchers contend that modifications preventing the development of these brain changes in younger and mid-life people could have a major impact on the incidence of the disease. Over the last two decades, a number of investigators and research groups have reported that adherence to a dietary pattern that includes fish but excludes red, organ, or processed meats is associated with a decreased risk of disease, while consumption of these meats and other items is linked with an increased risk. Although some remain skeptical, other research groups have conducted a number of human and animal tests that have verified this association and undertaken preliminary randomized long-term interventions targeting this construct.

2. The Role of Diet in Alzheimer's Prevention

Alzheimer's is the most common form of dementia—responsible for up to 80% of all cases of the disease in old age. However, it is not a normal part of aging. Like cardiovascular disease, Alzheimer's is thought to develop as a result of "the complex interplay of variables, including genetics, the environment, and lifestyle." In addition to cardiovascular disease and metabolic syndrome, inflammation, infection, genetics, head injury, depression and lower mood have been implicated as risk factors of Alzheimer's, although these connections are not as certain. Alternate or additional developing risk factors may be glue ear, malformations, autism spectrum disorders or other developmental disorders, and being born below 2.5 lbs (1.13 kg) or 5.5 lbs (2.49 kg). Dietary lifestyle choices can, however, support the immune system and ameliorate or potentiate moods irrespective of other risk factors.

It's not for naught that so much attention has been paid to Alzheimer's. Instead of losing the faculties that lend us to self-sufficiency, we lose those that lead us to forget who we are. Preventing this fate is paramount. And indeed, what we eat—and often when we eat—has been implicated in Alzheimer's risk. Diet, besides, affects cardiovascular disease, type 2 diabetes and its antecedent, metabolic syndrome. Each diagnosis has been correlated with an increased likelihood of dementia and decreased cognitive function. Alzheimer's is thought to be the confluence of all of these diseases, so it makes sense that we'd be interested in nutrition for its prevention.

Dietary strategies for slowing and preventing Alzheimer's disease The best diet for brain health

2.1. Nutrients and Compounds Linked to Brain Health

Many research studies have been conducted which provide the background for the development of the dietary guidelines for the AD-PREVENT study (Table 2), a follow-up trial to the FINGER Study that provides evidence for a multi-domain lifestyle intervention that involves diet, physical activity, and cognitive training plus cardiac risk factors for prevention of cognitive decline and dementia. In addition to a personalized diet, the guidelines recommend regular meals with a focus on lean proteins, plenty of plant-based foods, fermented foods, nuts, and good fats. Only a small amount of red meat and processed meats is recommended, and sweets are located in the "Use for special occasions or to treat yourself" group. They also recommend 4-6 servings of fruits and six of vegetables and day and half a cup of legumes as a protein source. Although the evidence for nutrient intake and relationship to cognitive decline or dementia is lean, one important finding from the Honolulu Asia Aging Study was that a high intake of antioxidants, such as vitamins C and E, was associated with better cognitive function in late life. This chapter will provide a summary of how dietary strategies may be employed over the life course to slow or prevent decline in cognitive function and the development of Alzheimer's disease.

The essentiality of many nutrients and their active compounds for brain health is relatively well established. Table 1 presents specific nutrients and their roles in cognitive function, sources in the diet, and the degree of scientific evidence for an association with cognition. This matrix was first published as a chapter in a book we edited in 2010 and was republished in 2013. Using strict criteria, which included only human studies published in English, over 800 studies with very specific web links were chosen that had been published in 2000 or later.

3. Popular Diets for Alzheimer's Prevention

The Ketogenic Diet works by forcing the body to use fat for energy instead of glucose. This is thought to be helpful to brain cells because not only can it reduce age-related inflammation, but it can also help in the survival of damaged cells. The Mediterranean and MIND Diets are effectively similar diets which focus on polyphenol-rich, antioxidant and anti-inflammatory foods. Reducing these pro-inflammatory foods can be damaging to the brain, especially for those who have the APOE4 gene variant. These diets encourage anti-inflammatory foods to help bolster these individuals. In addition, the Mediterranean Diet provides a moderate amount of wine. It is well known that red wine contains a good profile of polyphenols and antioxidants, including resveratrol, which seems to stimulate the brain to protect its cells by making its own antioxidants, always a better option than consuming commercially-available antioxidants.

High-profile public figures like Maria Shriver and Newt Gingrich have helped place Alzheimer's disease (AD) at the center of the national conversation on disease prevention and anti-aging. Various diets have shown potential as interventions to slow or prevent Alzheimer's, including the Ketogenic Diet, the Mediterranean Diet, and the MIND Diet. The Ketogenic Diet is a high-fat, moderate protein, and low-carbohydrate diet that requires the body to use fat for energy instead of glucose. The Mediterranean Diet prioritizes fruits and vegetables, whole grains, nuts, and olive oil with a moderate wine intake; and reduced consumption of red meat and refined flour. Similarly, the MIND diet encourages several servings of leafy greens and vegetables a week, berries 2x/week, beans every other day, 3 servings of whole grains a day, 1 oz raw nuts a day, fish once a week, a serving of poultry, 2 servings of berries a week, limited red meat, butter, and fast food. It also encourages 1 glass of wine a day.

3.1. Mediterranean Diet

Patients with Alzheimer's disease, a type of dementia, have three pathological hallmarks in their brains: senile plaques and neurofibrillary tangles documented by Alois Alzheimer himself in 1906, and recently chronic inflammation (or microgliosis), the latter possibly representing an auxiliary site to intervene for facilitating the reconstruction of lost synapses and to increase already poor neuroplasticity that characterizes Alzheimer's disease even in its early stages. Numerous scientific studies have shown that people who closely follow a Mediterranean diet have a low risk for Alzheimer's disease, the most common cause of dementia and chronic forgetfulness, where amyloid protein and a huge amount of this plaque are accumulated in the brains of patients. The diet can also help to prevent mild cognitive decline to severe dementia, and similar to the Mediterranean diet, it is designed to lower blood pressure, cholesterol, and blood sugar levels for heart and blood vessel disease.

3.1. Mediterranean Diet. The Mediterranean diet dates back to the 1950s, when it was first identified and described by science, and to 1995, when the first pyramid and its twelve food groups were proposed. It was the traditional diet of Greece and Southern Italy in the early 1960s, where adult life expectancy is some of the highest in the world, and rates of chronic disease among the lowest. A Spanish version of the Mediterranean diet pyramid was also proposed in 1999. Since that time, it has been shown that those who closely follow a Mediterranean diet are approximately 50% less likely to die from any cause, given that it is composed of healthy fats, lean proteins, antioxidants, and many anti-inflammatory foods.

4. Foods to Include in an Alzheimer's Prevention Diet

1. Foods Rich in Antioxidants: Blueberries, as well as other deeply colored fruits, are rich in antioxidants. Eating fruits and vegetables containing antioxidants is said to protect your brain cells, helping to prevent Alzheimer's. Fruit in particular has been found to help protect against plaque in your brain - the buildup of proteins that lead to Alzheimer's disease. Apples themselves contain quercetin, a potent antioxidant that has been found to protect against plaque in the brain. Vegetables containing antioxidants include carrots, red bell peppers, and avocados. 2. Foods High in Omega-3s: Fatty fish like salmon contain omega-3 fatty acids like docosahexaenoic acid (DHA) and eicosapentaenoic acid (EPA). Healthy fats like these are said to keep your memory sharp and mind alert as you age, helping to prevent Alzheimer's disease by reducing inflammation. Women who obtained higher intakes of ALA, though not EPA or DHA, when examining both dietary and supplement sources, showed higher test scores in studying, reading, and working on puzzles.

If you want to eat to protect your brain, a diet that emphasizes plant-based foods has been found to reduce your risk of cognitive decline. For example, eating a diet high in antioxidants has been found to improve cognitive function in adults, while fruits, vegetables, nuts, olive oil, and whole grains consumed following a heart-healthy diet plan have been found to reduce the overall risk or delay the onset of Alzheimer's disease. Several foods have also been found to potentially lower your risk of developing Alzheimer's all on their own. For example:

4.1. Fatty Fish and Omega-3 Fatty Acids

An observational study of 815 older adults reported that high fish consumption was associated with a lower risk of developing all-cause dementia, especially Alzheimer's, over 4–5 years. Clinical trials of fish oils that have found that they confer a cognitive improvement support their further development as a prevention treatment. However, it remains possible that the FDA may do an about-turn. The agents salsalate nor roflumilast also confer a cognitive enhancement and so it will be important to assess which, if any, of these candidate treatments confer an advantage in terms of dosing, side effects and other variables. More than a dozen observation studies have strongly suggested that eating fish once a week or more can result in a 50% reduced risk for developing Alzheimer's disease. The studies are less clear on what the best age might be to start the consumption of fish; the studies show the age of clinical dementia diagnosis was postponed regardless of ethnic group, personal history of stroke and presence or absence of the Alzheimer pathology. Some studies report a clear correlation of dietary fortification of 1000 mg of DHA per day to measurable improvement in cognitive function tests when compared to individuals whose daily intake of DHA was 500 mg or less.

Fatty fish (like salmon and mackerel), as well as the omega-3 fatty acids that they are rich in, have received a great deal of attention for their possible role in the prevention of Alzheimer's. The body of experimental work on omega-3 fatty acids primarily concerns candidate mechanisms linking them with Alzheimer's prevention. The two omega-3s of greatest interest are docosahexaenoic acid (DHA) and eicosapentaenoic acid (EPA). Both EPA and DHA have been found to confer anti-inflammatory and anti-oxidative effects. They are also both crucial components of cellular membranes in the brain. There is some evidence that DHA and EPA may also protect neurons through other mechanisms. Evidence from observational studies in humans is mixed. Cross-sectional studies have not consistently found that having raised erythrocyte or plasma DHA concentrations are associated with having a reduced risk of Alzheimer's disease, nor with having better clinical outcomes. The results of long-term studies of omega-3 fatty acids and cognitive outcomes in humans have, in contrast, where dietary intake of omega-3 fatty acids was measured prior to cognitive decline, been consistently positive. Furthermore, a number of short-term trials suggest that high-dose DHA supplementation can confer improvements in some, albeit not all, cognitive tests in healthy volunteers and in individuals with mild cognitive impairment.

4.1. Fatty Fish and Omega-3 Fatty Acids

4. ICMTS - Full-paper Dietary Strategies for Slowing and Preventing Alzheimer's Disease

5. Foods to Avoid in an Alzheimer's Prevention Diet

Saturated and trans fats. Diets high in saturated fat (the kind found in deep-fried fast food and animal protein) or trans fats (hydrogenated oils, margarine, and many packaged/processed foods, fast food) weaken arteries and raise the risk for cognitive impairment. Refined white sugars. In many studies, a high carbohydrate intake was linked to an increased risk for dementia, cognitive decline, and gallstones. A "sweeter" diet was associated with a smaller brain size, higher levels of insulin resistance, and a lower overall cognitive score. Sugars are inflammatory, metabolically inactive, and anti-nutrients that damage nerves and impede brain function. Toxic byproducts of animal protein's metabolism (especially beef and pork). When the body processes animal protein, harmful byproducts with noxious effects on the liver and brain are produced. Nitrosamines and advanced glycation end products (AGEs) are two of these toxic byproducts. Decreased levels of produced AGEs are linked to improvements in Alzheimer's disease symptoms. Swapping out consumption of red meat and processed pork items with fish and other non-meat sources of protein including beans, legumes, and nuts is a good idea.

Can certain dietary strategies slow down or completely prevent the progression of Alzheimer's disease? According to studies, that might actually be the case. It should come as no major surprise that some of the worst foods for the heart are also some of the worst foods for the brain. Empty calories, high amounts of saturated fat, high levels of cholesterol, and a variety of different toxins can help to impede brain function and thinking ability - which can, over time, increase the risk of developing Alzheimer's disease or other forms of cognitive decline.

5.1. Trans Fats and Saturated Fats

Saturated fatty acids (SFA) and cholesterol can accumulate in the brain over time and restrict cerebral blood flow, leading to neurodegeneration. They also adversely affect insulin signaling in the brain. Saturated fat given to animals before inducing Alzheimer's I created a sixteen hormone to protect his hormone from changes in the brain. We, as modern humans, do not have to consume any cholesterol to make sure to have the hormones that we need. Lard, butter, cheese, chicken meat, whole chicken, canned tuna, and fish, such as steelhead trout, salmon, and canned tuna all contribute substantial amounts of cholesterol to our diet and should be excluded from the diet for the purpose of Alzheimer's prevention.

Evidence exists that trans fats are a risk factor for AD, and those with a higher intake exhibit worse Alzheimer's disease, in general, suggesting that trans fats may promote the stress of brain aging. Additionally, a high intake of saturated fat may be particularly damaging to brain health in genetically predisposed individuals. An extensive evidence base links the consumption of both trans fats and saturated fats to the development of AD. In Alzheimer's disease, there is a negative association between saturated and trans fats with brain size and learning and memory. The sources of saturated and trans fats that are most potentially a risk factor for developing Alzheimer's disease include beef, veal, pork, lamb, poultry, added butter, fat, and added shortening. It is important to eliminate these foods from our diet to reduce Alzheimer's risk and promote brain health.

6. Meal Planning and Recipes for Brain Health

Menu and Recipes components This document focuses on the dietary pattern and other lifestyle factors that have been shown to be most consistently linked to slowing and preventing AD. The dietary pattern that was reviewed is the "STOP-AD diet." This diet is similar to some other healthy dietary patterns and can be adapted to vegan and vegetarian needs. The nutrition information was reviewed by. Portions of Life Plan were reviewed by the American Brain Foundation (ABF) and retained by ABF. The ABF can provide CME and CEU credit in the future. Recipes are protected by copyright and may not be copied, printed, or shared without written consent from the American Brain Foundation. Support to create the recipes was provided by the VanAuken Foundation and Drexel University.

Why do you need a meal plan? 4 out of 5 (or 2.5 million) older Americans have multiple chronic conditions, with their healthcare consuming 66% of the US healthcare system. Brain health is a critical aspect of overall health and thus has a significant impact on this system. Our brain health results indicate the extent to which we can remain free of dementia and have the cognitive abilities to promote independence and the capability to carry out activities of daily living. Diet has also been linked to slowing cognitive decline and reducing the risk of AD. Thus, being able to plan meals with components from a special dietary pattern will likely be of great interest.

Meal Planning & Recipes for Brain Health

Dinner Meatless chili made with kidney beans sautéed in onions, green onions, red and green bell peppers, with added mushrooms and diced tomatoes, and seasoned with chili powder, oregano, and ground black pepper ½ cup quinoa or brown rice served with the chili.

Snack 1 apple ½ cup of edamame shelled and cooked in 1-2 teaspoons of olive oil with curry powder

Lunch Old-fashioned or steel-cut oats cooked with powdered cinnamon and nutmeg for an extra anti-inflammatory kick. If you like, stir in ¼-1/2 cup of frozen blueberries and let it sit for a few minutes before you eat. When you stir, the creamy color of the oats will turn a beautiful lavender due to the interaction of the blueberries with the antioxidants in those spices. A hearty dose of healthy fats, served on the side of 0%-fat Greek yogurt

Breakfast 2-egg, spinach, onion, and mushroom omelet served with salsa for an extra anti-inflammatory boost ½ piece of whole grain toast spread with either all-natural peanut butter or almond butter

One Day Meal Plan

To pull all of these concepts together, I'll translate the dietary strategies into a sample meal plan. This meal plan will include lean protein, including at least one serving of seafood, vegetables and fruit in every meal, healthy fats, nuts, legumes, whole grains, and resistant starches to support gut health. Spices will be used liberally, with an extra emphasis on food anti-inflammation, telling specifically which spices to use and why they're so good for the brain.

7. Conclusion and Future Directions

By focusing on preventing the onset and progression of Alzheimer's, we can reduce the suffering that results from this disease and reduce the burden it places on health and social care services. In the future, we will need to conduct large-scale interventional trials to test the effect of a number of dietary components. This will probably involve using a composite score based on routinely available information related to diet: the indices described earlier. As we have seen, these indices are based on diet guidelines for the general public; this is important given the difficulty in changing the dietary habits of a great number of individuals.

Overall, it is clear that dietary strategies for preventing or slowing cognitive decline are still in the relatively early stages in comparison to the more established lines of research exploring pharmacological and lifestyle interventions. However, the increasing rates of cognitive impairment mean that it is more important than ever to try to explore as many potential avenues as possible. Diet has been associated with cognitive function in cross-sectional studies, and recent large-scale longitudinal studies have suggested protective roles for consumption of some dairy and whole-grain products; some protective effects have also been observed for a Mediterranean-style diet. High levels of fat and sugar are generally thought to be associated with poor cognitive function and cognitive decline, while intake of some nutrients and vitamins may protect against cognitive decline. It is important, however, that we continue to explore the many potentially modifiable risk factors, including diet, which may slow the rate of cognitive decline or, more importantly, prevent cognitive decline becoming clinically relevant.

www.ingramcontent.com/pod-product-compliance
Lightning Source LLC
Chambersburg PA
CBHW070825260726

48660CB00005B/1999